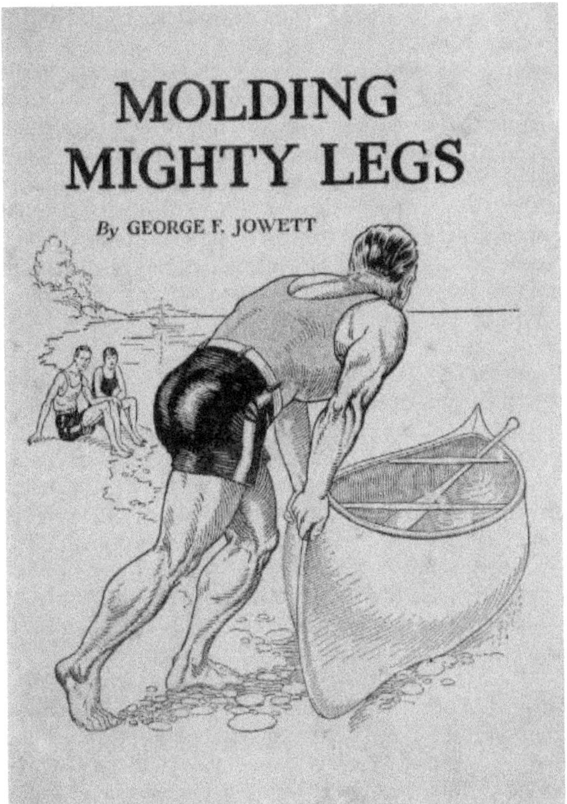

MOLDING MIGHTY LEGS

By GEORGE F. JOWETT

The information contained in this publication is for historical and educational purposes only and is not designed to and does not provide medical, nutritional, or health advice, diagnosis, or opinion for any health or individual problem. The material presented is not a substitute for medical or other professional health services from a qualified health care provider who is familiar with the unique facts of the individual, and should not be used in place of a visit, call, consultation, or advice of a physician or other healthcare provider. Individuals should always consult a qualified health care provider about any health concern and prior to undertaking any new treatment. The publisher assumes no responsibility and specifically disclaims all liability for any consequence relating directly or indirectly to any action or inaction that a reader takes based on any information contained herein.

Be advised that no one should undertake exercises in the nature of those addressed in this book without prior consultation with a physician. Nor does the publisher make any representations concerning whether any of the exercises or suggestions provided by the trainers or physical fitness specialists featured in this book would be effective or appropriate for the reader's needs or expectations. The publisher expressly disclaims any and all responsibility and/or liabilities that might result from the uninformed or misinformed application of the techniques identified herein as well as for any unsupervised physical fitness training.

Finally, the publisher disclaims any and all liabilities arising from the use of any equipment featured in this book and makes no representations as to the utility, safety, or adequacy of the equipment generally or with respect to any specific purpose.

MOLDING
MIGHTY LEGS
(ORIGINAL VERSION, RESTORED)

By

GEORGE F. JOWETT

Original Publisher: The Jowett Institute of Physical
Culture, 422 Poplar Street, Scranton, P.A., 1931.

PUBLISHED BY O'Faolain Patriot LLC, Copyright
2011

info@PhysicalCultureBooks.com

ISBN-13: 978-1466476752

ISBN-10: 1466476753

Published in the United States of America

To Order More Copies Visit: Physical
Culture Books.com

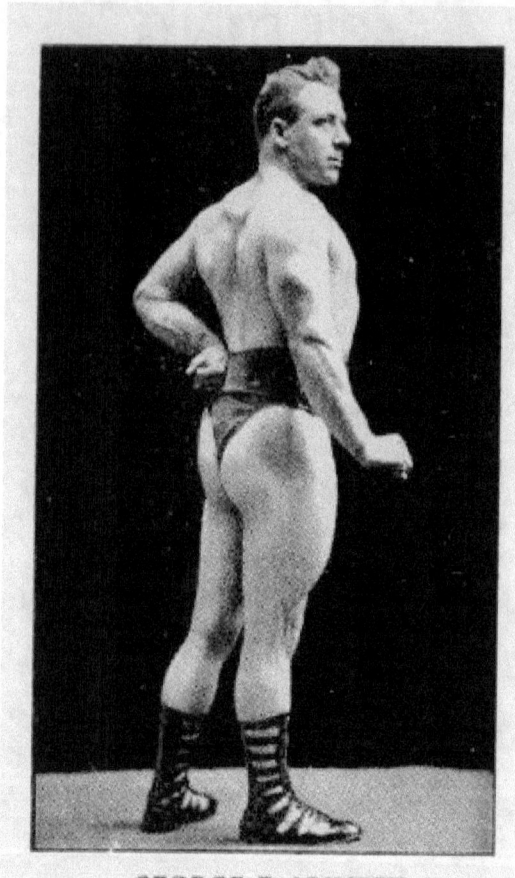

GEORGE F. JOWETT

Champion of Champions

THE STORY OF GEORGE F. JOWETT

THE story of George F. Jowett is most inspiring to all who are seeking great strength and a powerfully developed body. As a boy he was badly injured and physicians declared he would never live to see the age of fifteen. What the physicians overlooked was the consuming flame of desire which burned within the weak, undersized body. His heart's desire, like that of everyone who lacks physical perfection, was to possess a body, big, vibrant, and powerful. How he overcame his physical problems and rose to be one of the world's strongest and best- built athletes reads like a romance.

He won his way to become Champion of Champions because he believed in clean living and exercise. The fact that he had to fight for what he got places him in a better position to understand how the other fellow feels. He knows what has to be faced and, backed by his great experience and tremendous enthusiasm for helping others, he has made thousands of weaklings into magnificent specimens of vital, glorious manhood. Dr. Bernard in his story, "The March of a Great Athlete," eulogizes George F. Jowett as the finest example of physical manhood—an example to be imitated and followed.

Making others like himself is George F. Jowett's life hobby. It is a passion with him. He would love to make every man better than himself if it were possible. His heart is in the right place and the man who accepts him for his own teacher makes a splendid choice.

From a bed of sickness to the throne of Champion of Champions is his story. He made his own body mighty with big, shapely, powerful muscles. No physical problem of yours is a problem to him. He holds the answers and gives them to you as you want them. In him you have a teacher who is an athlete from the crown of his head to the soles of his feet—one who does by deeds and not by words. If you want to succeed get him for your teacher. If you want big muscles, a shapely body, tons of energy, and great strength with inexhaustible endurance sign your enrolment with the Champion of Champions and you will surely succeed.

MOLDING MIGHTY LEGS
By GEORGE F. JOWETT

THE development of the lower limbs is probably the greatlyest problem a body builder has to face. Only too often does he see the legs remain unchanged no matter what he does, while the body, from the waist up, develops pleasing proportions. The result is the exerciser becomes, at best, only a half-built man.

The degree of disappointment arising from this unbalanced condition is often very keen. Many have written to me and said they would give anything if they could only get one inch of growth on each calf. I know just how embarrassing the situation can be because I also have been through the mill. I was not always as well built as I am now and as I have been for a number of years. Even when I was very strong and powerfully built "upstairs," my lower limbs spoiled the picture. Although I was able to build good thighs yet my calf measurement at one time could only show a meager 14^-inch circumference when at the same time my upper arm measured 16£ inches and I had a 45-inch chest—my thighs then were 24 inches.

I tried everything to make the calf muscles grow, also I sought the advice of every well known authority of that time. They questioned me and when they found out I had done all the exercises they were familiar with and had followed many other methods they were not then acquainted with, the only consolation offered was "nature never intended me to have larger calves and nothing I could do would improve them." I guess they all thought I was a physical culture atheist because I refused to accept their consolation. I argued that life is growth, and muscle is life which the unchangeable law of nature controls by its daily process of breaking down and building up. The muscles of the legs are composed of no different structure than other muscles, except that they are denser in structure. I further argued that there must be a way which, if no one else was able to inform me of, I would find out for myself.

Like all enthusiastic body builders I yearned to be a heavyweight. The fact that I was lauded as the strongest middleweight ever known did not interest me. I believed in the old proverb that "A good little man could never beat a good big man" and— perhaps like you—I wished to be a good big man. I firmly believed if I could solve the leg problem I would hold the solution of transforming myself into a heavyweight, filling my body with greater strength as I increased all my proportions. How truly this belief became a fact is recalled by all who know me as a powerfully-built middleweight. Remarkable though it may seem, still it is a fact that after I had reached the years of maturity I astonished the physical culture world by developing my calves from 14£ inches until they had the massive circumference of 18£ inches. As they increased in growth so did every other bodily measurement

8

until I developed from what experts claimed to be a perfect physical specimen of 154 lbs. stripped, into a perfect physical specimen of 200 lbs. stripped.

I am reciting this experience for your benefit, because my success in body growth has always been looked upon as an interesting and phenomenal experience. These facts will also give you courage to keep striving because it is a well established fact that a man who has acquired great muscular proportions and strength for his height will find it more difficult to increase body growth. The peculiar part is, no other teacher has been able to advance any new training methods to take care of the legs. In other words, little has been added to what was known about leg building years ago. You would be amazed if you could see the lower limb development of 99% of physical training teachers—their lower limb development is so poor.

Bearing all this in mind I believe when you have finished reading this treatise you will be well satisfied that you have learned something entirely new in leg building and something that will enable you to get busy and get bigger and better legs.

First you have to know something about the muscular formation of the body from the hips down to the ground and what their special functions are. It really is amazing to find as we go lower down from the hips to the sole of the foot how numerous the muscles become and what an amazing influence better leg construction has upon the upper body, particularly upon the organs.

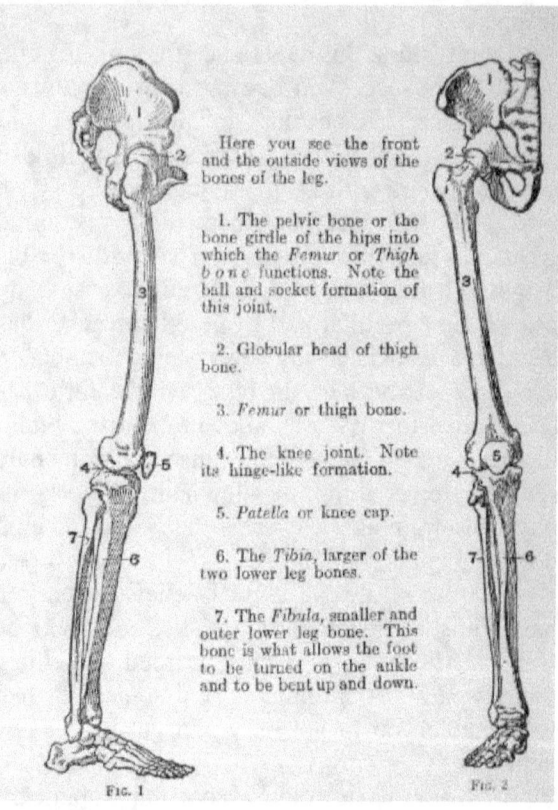

Here you see the front and the outside views of the bones of the leg.

1. The pelvic bone or the bone girdle of the hips into which the *Femur* or *Thigh bone* functions. Note the ball and socket formation of this joint.

2. Globular head of thigh bone.

3. *Femur* or thigh bone.

4. The knee joint. Note its hinge-like formation.

5. *Patella* or knee cap.

6. The *Tibia*, larger of the two lower leg bones.

7. The *Fibula*, smaller and outer lower leg bone. This bone is what allows the foot to be turned on the ankle and to be bent up and down.

FIG. 1   FIG. 2

The skeleton of the lower limbs swings on, or depends from the pelvic girdle, which is the bony section of the hips. (See Figs. 1 and 2.) The globular head of the thigh bone is fastened into the hip joint rather tightly like a ball and socket joint. It is the formation of the thigh joint into the hip that gives the leg its rotary action. It is generally conceded, that men with wide hips have strong, well-proportioned legs.

MUSCULAR STRUCTURE

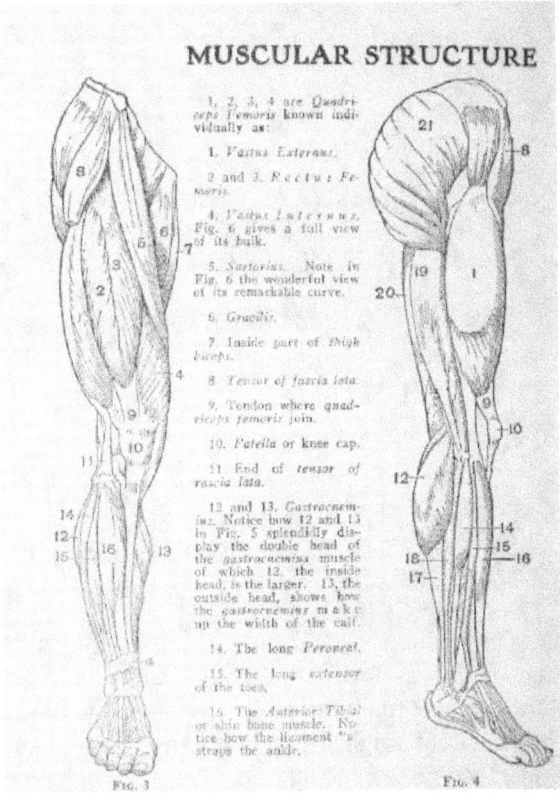

1, 2, 3, 4 are *Quadriceps Femoris* known individually as:

1. *Vastus Externus.*

2 and 3. *Rectus Femoris.*

4. *Vastus Internus,* Fig. 6 gives a full view of its bulk.

5. *Sartorius.* Note in Fig. 6 the wonderful view of its remarkable curve.

6. *Gracilis.*

7. Inside part of *thigh biceps.*

8. *Tensor of fascia lata.*

9. Tendon where *quadriceps femoris* join.

10. *Patella* or knee cap.

11. End of *tensor of fascia lata.*

12 and 13. *Gastrocnemius.* Notice how 12 and 13 in Fig. 5 splendidly display the double head of the *gastrocnemius* muscle of which 12, the inside head, is the larger. 13, the outside head, shows how the *gastrocnemius* make up the width of the calf.

14. The long *Peroneal.*

15. The long *extensor* of the toes.

16. The *Anterior Tibial* or shin bone muscle. Notice how the ligament "s" straps the ankle.

Fig. 3   Fig. 4

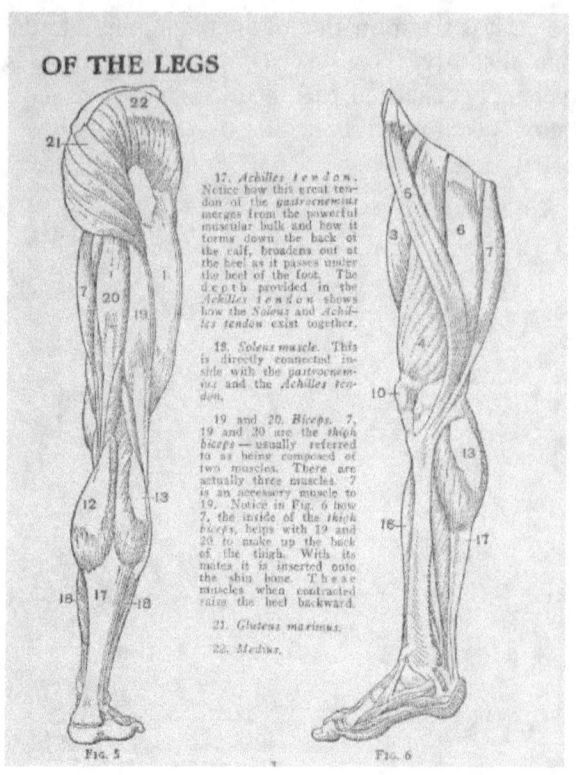

17. *Achilles tendon.* Notice how this great tendon of the *gastrocnemius* merges from the powerful muscular bulk and how it forms down the back of the calf, broadens out at the heel as it passes under the heel of the foot. The depth provided in the *Achilles tendon* shows how the *Soleus* and *Achilles tendon* exist together.

18. *Soleus muscle.* This is directly connected inside with the *gastrocnemius* and the *Achilles tendon.*

19 and 20. *Biceps.* 7, 19 and 20 are the *thigh biceps* — usually referred to as being composed of two muscles. There are actually three muscles. 7 is an accessory muscle to 19. Notice in Fig. 6 how 7, the inside of the *thigh biceps,* helps with 19 and 20 to make up the back of the thigh. With its mates it is inserted onto the shin bone. These muscles when contracted raise the heel backward.

21. *Glutens maximus.*

22. *Medius.*

Fig. 5   Fig. 6

Personally, I would not say this is altogether true as far as the entire leg is concerned, for although a broad-hipped person usually has a good pair ot thighs, this holds true only in the upper region of the crotch. The leg, only too often, tapers off quickly toward the knee showing no development of the internus vastus muscle which is located just above the inside of the knee. Still the broad-hipped man, similar to a man with wide shoulders, has the heavier framework to build on. A wide pelvis will invariably be coupled with a thigh bone which is a little thicker than the average.

Years ago the perfect specimen of manhood was supposed to have wide shoulders and narrow hips and legs of the greyhound type. How ridiculous that is we now well know. A broad-shouldered man should have hips of almost equal circumference. Broad hips should be a sign of great leg strength. Men of this type are usually very virile and energetic. But, whether a man be wide-hipped, or narrow, he will have to make the decision as to whether his "pendulums of propulsion" will be props of power or like a pair of weak hinges. They can be either—depending on his decision.

It may surprise you to learn that one lower limb, not including the pelvis, has thirty bones in its makeup. Naturally these bones are all subject to articulation, or movement, and that can only be accomplished by the influence of muscles. Most people have the idea there are only two muscles in the legs—the thigh and the calf. In the average leg it looks that way, but when we start the job of leg building we find it very different. Still we are only going to deal with the important muscles— which are plenty —as many of the other muscles are minor or accessory muscles and therefore act as "helping" muscles to the larger muscles.

The largest muscle is the one that bulks on the front of the thigh known as the quadriceps femoris, meaning "the four-fold thigh muscle."

This is sometimes incorrectly known as the triceps jemoris, but don't get confused with these two names. Triceps means three-fold, which is an erroneous title to apply to these muscles, as there are actually four. The most important of this group are the two divisions of the rectus femoris and the two vastus muscles which we shall deal with separately. In connection with this discussion of the muscles of the leg see Figs. 3, 4, 5, and 6. In Fig. 3 you will observe that these four muscles join one common tendon, marked 9 in the illustration.

The rectus femoris is the largest and lies directly on the front of the thigh, It begins from the hip bone close to where the hip socket is bulking heavily and descends to end a short distance above the knee where it joins the common tendon along with the other muscles. The action of this muscle is to straighten the leg. This being the case it is necessary that this muscle be very strong. As it develops, the front of the thigh becomes round and bulks from a little below the hip to about four inches above the knee. Just stiffen the knee and you will see where this muscle ends.

The full contour of the upper thigh is not given by this or any of the other muscles of the quadriceps group. Another muscle, which I will discuss later, bulks above where the rectus femoris begins and contributes to this scheme, filling out the extreme upper thigh; it tapers off into a very long tendon running on the extreme outside of the leg flat against the vastus externus.

This last-named muscle, the vastus externus, arises from the upper femur Done—which is the thigh bone—and has a convex appearance. It comprises the outside contour of the thigh, meeting the outer posterior muscle of the back of the thigh and also presses against the margin of the rectus femoris. The fibers of this muscle, as they near the knee, pass into a flat tendon before it joins the common tendon which goes to the knee.

The two muscles, rectus femoris and vastus externus, are ordinarily the best developed of the thigh—from natural causes. The rectus femoris is the more easily developed and the vastus externus almost as easily. Still they are rarely built to the proportions which nature would term average and are seldom adequate to meet any unusual daily effort. Just prove it. Walk up a number of steps slowly and you will quickly get out of breath.

Walking is advised as being one of the best forms of exercise for these two muscles, but I certainly do not subscribe to that belief. In the first place we have seen that these leg muscles have to do mostly with erection—that is, straightening the legs. This straightening should take place as the leg goes forward and when it straightens under the weight of the body, but how many people actually straighten the leg in a manner to give full contraction to these erector muscles? Very few. The average man walks loose kneed and walks from the knees. Women walk mostly from the hips, and on the average they have a better- shaped leg than has a man. The man who takes a long stride, steps out from the hip. He gets the full double extension and contraction of these muscles. A man who walks vigorously, while not necessarily with a long stride, obtains strong femoris contraction as the leg stiffens under the pelvis to supply the vigorous forward propulsion of the body.

Climbing produces a splendid development of these muscles, but is exhausting if the muscles on the back of the thigh are not developed in proportion. Climbing also has a reaction upon the heart, especially if the leg muscles are not balanced. No doubt you have often climbed a steep grade, or many steps, and found if you immediately began to descend your legs trembled and the knees and thighs were weak. Sometimes this happens to such an extent that the support of a rail or a stick will be helpful.

The rectus femoris and vastus extemus are also the kicking muscles and are always found powerfully developed on the leg of a football player. They also act strongly in forward lunging movements. Stand alongside of a package case about five feet square and about 300 lbs. in weight and upend it. If you stand too closely, the effort will be all upon the arms and shoulders, and you will find it a tough job, but stand back with the right leg diagonally straight and the left leg bent forward at the Irnee and the arms held straight in front and you will find it 100% easier as the legs get into action and, being stronger than either your back or arms, they accomplish the trick with ease.

Watch a man accustomed to handling packing cases and you will see him handle it the way I say. He will also lower the body so he can get under the weight, so to speak, and thereby obtain greater power from the legs. This is an example where the muscles of the front of the thigh and the muscles of the back combine to perform an effort of resistance. If you were placed in a position that compelled you to support a weight across the shoulders—not lift or upend it—you would do better by keeping the feet in line with each other and the knees locked. The moment you bend the knees your leg strength will decrease and no matter how strong your arms and upper body are they will not help much to regain the first position of leg rigidity.

It has been generally said that weight lifters are all top heavy like hand balancers. To a certain extent it is true, but the strongest men in the world have powerful legs. Incidentally, I have found on investigation that the majority of these men were naturally equipped with big strong legs. In other words, they never were called upon to worry about leg development. But the fellow who has only ordinary development finds that by lifting weights his upper body develops out of all proportion to his lower limbs, and very little gain will his legs acquire, no matter how much deep knee bending he does. When practicing the deep knee bending exercises you generally see him struggling with a weight across his shoulders that is just about all he can support. Every squat he makes is a strain. He holds his breath and winds up breathing very hard. In this exercise there is a great strain imposed upon the upper body in striving to control the weight. So much so that the heart finds it hard to supoly body and legs with sufficient blood fuel with the result that the compression in the lungs stifles stimulation. It generally happens that more harm than good is done, and the disappointing part is the legs remain about the same in size. I have seen exercise fans struggle with this exercise until their eyes were distended from the head, and the veins stood out as though they would burst. How can any sane, thinking person believe any good can come out of such a terrible practice? I have seen, and so have you, many fellows with powerful-looking arms, back and chest, fail miserably when attempting to carry a load on their backs. When it is shouldered they simply cannot move. If they do move then- knees fold up like weak hinges. So, no matter how strong your upper body is, unless the legs are also strong, they will not be able to back up your bodily effort.

Arthur Saxon always claimed the most important muscle in the thigh is the vastus internus—the inside thigh member of the quadriceps femoris. This muscle displays its prominence directly above the inside of the knee in a short chunky mound. The great importance of this muscle is its rock-like power in locking the knee. In this operation it bulges out boldly, but when the knee is bent it loses its fulness. Acting together these four divisions of the quadriceps femoris—the two parts of the rectus femoris, the vastus externus and the vastus internus extend the leg on the thigh.

A little earlier in this book I said that the quadriceps femoris did not provide the entire outer or upper front contour of the thigh. High up in the pelvis a muscle, the tensor of the fascia lata, arises and fills in the gap helping to complete that beautiful outside sweeping curve seen on a well-developed thigh. Its muscle structure is short, then tapers away into a long band-like tendon down the outside of the thigh. In Fig. 3 the artist purposely cut it off so the vastus externus could be better seen. However, he did not dispense with any of the muscle structure. From the end cutoff it runs down in a long ribbon tendon alongside of the vastus externus and becomes inserted on the outside of the calf bone just below the knee. This is an important feature and aids the vastus externus considerably in raising the leg sidewise.

The muscles of the legs that draw the legs together from the knees spread-apart position we call the gracilis. Hollowed-out thighs on the inside are the result of poor gracilis development. The muscle, as its name explains, is a slim, slender strip arising from the pelvic bone to fasten on the shin bone just below the inside of the knee.

The other important thigh muscle that originates from the pelvis and fastens below the knee is the sartorius. This is the longest muscle in the body and is a very interesting and unusual

19

member of thigh construction. The word sartorius is Latin, meaning "to mend." Early anatomists took the meaning to be "tailor's muscle" because of the position the tailor sits in to mend garments. The Germans regard it as the "cutting" muscle because it cuts across the other front thigh muscles commencing from the front outside edge of the hip, sweeping inward and downward in a big curve round to the inside of the knee to become fastened on the inside of the shin bone. If you hold your leg out in front with a slightly bent knee and twist the thigh out on the hip joint the sartorius will spring into prominence. It will then be firm and tense as it will be doing the most of the work of holding the leg in this awkward position. The sartorius acts as a binding strap to the quadriceps femoris in the same manner as a hoop straps a barrel.

Now you have an idea of what the muscles on the front, the inside and outside of the leg do, consequently you will see immediately that simply making a deep knee bend is not sufficient to develop all the muscles on the front and sides of the thigh, though the deep knee bend is often given as the best all around thigh exercise.

The other important thigh muscles are those located at the back of the thigh. (See Fig. 5.) These are known as the biceps —meaning, as does the arm biceps, the Twin head muscles. Actually there are three muscles in this group and they are referred to for study as three hamstring muscles. Their action is to flex the knee, that is, bend it, and also to raise the leg backward. These muscles are undoubtedly the poorest developed in the thigh of the average body builder. They should be cultivated, not only because of the balanced strength they give to the leg, but because of the beautiful appearance they provide when viewing the thigh from the side. They give a fulness similar to a half moon curve and display their great strength and contour when the heel is drawn up and back on the thigh. I have seen but very few who possess this shapely curve, but those who display it most are short-distance runners—the hundred-yard man. It is a great forward-driving muscle while the front muscles are great thrusting muscles.

Did you ever try to raise your leg and hold it at right angles with the body without bending back? Try, by holding on to the back of a chair, and you will see that the leg cannot be brought horizontally before you. It is a singular characteristic of the hamstring muscles that they are too short to permit full flexion on the thigh in the manner mentioned, but bend the knee and at once the thigh can be fully flexed past the horizontal position. The whole matter is that the much too short tendons are attached to the leg bones in such a way as to prevent the limb from moving any farther. As the knee is bent the points of attachment are brought closer together which immediately shortens the distance and relaxes the strain upon the hamstring tendons. The seat of insertion of these muscles is not upon the thigh bone, but upon the lower leg bones of the knee. People with bow-legged or knock-kneed

21

conditions generally are so because one of the hamstring tendons is contracted more than the others. Sometimes the condition is caused by the gracilis muscles, sometimes by the vastus externus, and as these muscles are developed the legs straighten.

I have helped many to overcome bow-legged conditions as well as knock-knees by a simple system of leg exercise. Leg braces are of no use at all. Mechanically they may straighten the leg some, but that does not improve the tendinous or muscular condition. Exercise is the surest remedy for permanent correction.

You will remember a little earlier in this discussion I remarked that most weight lifters are top heavy. I have proved this to them often by proving, to their surprise, that they are able to lift more weight to arms' length overhead, in a slow movement involving actual strength, while sitting on a chair than they were able to do when standing ud. This proves their upper body was developed more than the lower limbs, which should not be. Actually, it should be the reverse, as the leg muscles, being the largest in the body, naturally should have more strength. This being true, the lower limbs will easily give support to anything the upper body is capable of doing. In other words, a man should build his legs in greater proportion to his body than is usually done. Hand balancers and Roman Ring performers, like weight lifters, develop the same condition of top heaviness, while jumpers, pole vaulters and association football players develop legs in excess of that needed to balance their upper body development.

Now before we finish this thigh discussion I wish to draw to your attention one thing more that is not well known. Most people believe that their height is governed by the length of the spine, but this is not actually true. It is the length of the thigh bones that counts most. If these are short a man will never be tall and no amount of spine stretching will lengthen them for him. I wish to impress this on your mind, particularly if you are short in stature and anxious to increase your height. Many people have been seriously injured using machines to stretch the spine and at the most only got an inch increase.

Men with thigh bones longer than the bones of the shin have a longer running stride than those with shorter thigh bones. Successful sprinters, more so than long distance runners, usually have thigh bones longer than their shin bones. Also, runners in general and jumpers have wonderfully clean-cut knees. I do not know of anything that will set off the appearance of a pair of legs better than clean-cut knees and ankles. Some people naturally have thick, meaty knees and ankles. In the knees it is generally caused by an accumulation of fat, although people with poor blood stimulation have thick knees.

You will remember I mentioned each muscle of the quadriceps femoris joins the common tendon in the region of the knee. To be exact this takes place just above the knee, but this tendon descends and passes over the knee to become inserted on the shin bone below the knee. In this process it passes from a tendinous condition into that of a ligament and is known as the ligament of the patella. The patella is the knee cap or knee pan and is imbedded into the gristly tissue of the tendon. The real object of the knee cap is to act as a pulley to give greater power to the quadriceps femoris. Bearing this in mind you can readily see why weak thigh muscles are the cause of weak trembling knees. The more powerful the thigh muscles are the thicker is the knee tendon, therefore, the more securely seated is the knee cap and less danger is there of a twisted knee or a slipping knee cap.

It is interesting to know that absence of the normal supply of fat pellets and the amount of lubrication in the knee sac is what causes knee stitffness and knee cracking when the knee is bent forcibly. Uric acid in the blood seems to find the knee sectors a happy hunting ground. Anyhow such acid in the blood greatly affects the lubricating sources of the knee. Parasites in the blood strive to make inroads there and the absorption of the fatty substance of lubrication is what helps to bring about rheumatism. Consequently, clean-cut knees will not only reward you in leg shapeliness, but will add materially to your health.

Nature considers the knee a very important section. It is powerfully supported by thick flat ligaments and tendons which stabilize equilibrium by the various check ligaments that exist there. If you stand with the feet apart, but in line with each other, and look overhead and lean sharply back, you will instantly feel a lifting of the knee cap as the big knee tendon tenses under contraction of the thigh muscles as they function to preserve your balance. This will give you a good idea of the pulley action ol the patella ligament as it lifts and relaxes.

And now let us travel a little lower down to the calf itselt-- which thousands of body builders have named "the toughest part of the body to build." It really is all that and is due mostly to the fact that all the lower limb muscles lack the bulk of other muscles, excepting of course the muscle that forms on the back of the calf. The length of all the other calf muscles runs mostly to ligaments which act as powerful levers to all foot action. These ligaments are thick and tough and the muscle head of each has a structure which is remarkably closely woven (usually termed as being dense). It is well to remember that this condition alone makes muscle building of the lower limb very difficult. It is harder to break down the old tissue in order to create replacement and again the average foot action is not such as normally lends itself to the breaking down process. People who have shin bones shorter than their thigh bones are apt to have a pretty good calf development. This does not always mean they possess a larger measured calf, but it does mean that the calf will always show off better with development they are able to acquire. The muscle that is accumulated will bulk more largely on the calf because of the shorter area. Size and length of the foot have a great deal to do with appearance. A man who has a size ten foot will have to build a much bigger calf circumference in order to look well, than will a man with a size six foot.

Flat feet and long heels are unnatural difficulties to the leg developer, but they are problems which do occur, and which exercise will offset.

A long foot has the poorest toe grip. Normally the man with a short foot should have a better toe grip, but on the short foot the toe grip does not always come up to expectations. When the leg builder begins to wake up to the importance of developing a strong toe grip he will be somewhat astonished to realize the bearing this has upon the muscles of the calf.

The largest muscles on the calf are those which form the bulk on the back of the lower leg. These are known as the gastrocnemius muscles and have a double head. If you raise yourself high upon the toes you will notice a cleft in their bulk about the middle of the calf. This cleft is the dividing mark between the inner and outer heads of the gastrocnemius. These twin muscles arise separately from the back of the thigh bone just above the knee and quickly merge into closer association forming the main bulk, then taper off to become inserted into the heel bone through the intermediary membrane of the leg which is known as the Achilles tendon. Viewing the calf muscle from the back of the leg there is a perceptible break in the contour where the fleshy fibers are succeeded by the Achilles tendon. In a poorly developed leg there will be no break seen at all. The duty of the gastrocnemius is to extend the foot by pulling up on the heel bone and also in bringing the foot in a straight line with the leg. When acting alone the gastrocnemius is an accessary flexor of the leg on the thigh. It is this muscle that holds your bodily poise when standing on the toes and is a powerful driving muscle. The next time you see any hundred-yards sprinter in action observe how powerfully these muscles are employed in driving the body ahead. You do not see this nearly as well on the leg of a long distance runner, because he runs mostly on the flat of his foot, while the sprinter is bounding ahead upon the ball of his foot.

Connected with the gastrocnemius muscles is the Soleus muscle. It begins where the gastrocnemius leaves off to join the Achilles tendon. As you look at a well-shaped calf from the back of the leg you will notice right under the gastrocnemius a body of tissue which tapers in a broad triangle-shape toward the ankle. This is mainly the Soleus. Toward the ankle the Achilles is more evident as it runs to its heel-bone insertion. This threefold combination produces a result both extraordinary and powerful in the way they work together supporting each other in the great work of propelling your body weight forward.

There are only two direct foot movements—the straightening of the foot on the leg and the bending of the foot on the ankle upward, which takes place as the foot is advanced prior to placing on the ground in the stride. The muscle that functions this is the Anterior tibial, better known as the shin bone muscle. When developed it fills the calf out on the front outside, giving that pleasing smooth rounding to the outside of the calf. If you bend the foot upward, then rotate the foot on the ankle outward, this muscle will stand out in greater prominence. It arises on the outside of the front calf just below the knee and displays all its bulk on the outside, then merges into a strong thick tendon crossing the ankle to the inside of the foot where it continues to its seat of insertion under the arch of the foot.

Do not forget there are two bones in the lower leg just as in the forearm though the second bone is much smaller than the shin bone. This smaller bone provides the rotary action of the foot on the ankle by the muscular attachment which lodges there and inserts onto the toes. The big toe is favored by having a separate muscle of its own, named the great toe exterior. It arises about half way down on the outer of the two calf bones.

The Peroneus Tertius is a bigger muscle which helps to build up the outside bulk of the calf. It commences just below the knee and when it reaches the ankle branches off fanwise into four tendons which are fastened on the four toes.

The long Peroneal forms the direct outside of the calf arising from just below the knee and descending almost squarely until it reaches the ankle where it takes on a separate and rather unusual form. It branches into a long tendon passing right under and across the arch of the foot to fasten on the base of the great toe. The latter action is what turns the sole of the foot outwardly. The short Peroneal merges with the long Peroneal about half way down the latter. It also passes onto the sole of the foot to fasten on the little toe where it helps in foot extension. There are a number of superficial muscles but they are subject to the action of the muscles just mentioned except what are known as the short extensors of the toes. They arise from a short flat muscle right under the outside of the ankle, then branch off into four tendinous slips into the second, third, fourth, and great toe. This muscle is almost destroyed on the female foot by women who wear high-heeled shoes.

The muscles on the front and outside of the lower limb, as you will now realize, are all connected or inserted with the toes and the sole of the foot. This fact will clarify my statement of "the sooner leg builders realize the significance of the toe grip, the better results will be gotten." You will also understand why people who suffer from fallen arches and flat feet always have poor frontal and lateral muscular development. You will have seen why placing pressure on one or the other side of the foot or turning the foot in or out or pressing the toes strongly on the floor creates different leg muscular action which stimulates growth. Most leg builders do not see the difference between raising themselves on the toes of a straight-foot and raising themselves when the foot is turned acutely in or out—possibly because it has never been properly explained to them. People who have weak ankles, fallen arches, or flat feet should cultivate seriously the frontal and lateral muscles of the lower leg. If it were possible to get people to take about two dozen drop kicks at a football daily there would be no weak ankles or fallen arches. Still there are other easier and more convenient methods that are just as good.

The greatest error among leg builders is their utter lack of balance when performing leg exercises. Strange as it may seem, yet it is a fact that few perform correctly the common exercise of raising upon the toes while standing stiff-kneed. The object in this exercise is to make the muscles of the leg, particularly the gastrocnemius, lift the body weight up. Usually they teter up and down like a rocker under motion. If you stood any one of these haphazard exercisers alongside of an upright stick you would see at the conclusion of the exercises that their head and shoulders would be advanced about ten inches forward; but, make them keep their position perpendicular with the stick in a slow up-lifting movement and they quickly find a difference. Many are too lazy to raise themselves to the limit upon the toes. When they do, they usually complain of a cramp in the arch of the foot or the gastrocnemius muscles. Little do they seem to realize that the cramp is telling them only too plainly how badly the muscles are in need of just that muscular stimulation.

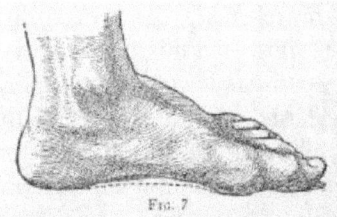

The finished drawing shows how a well-built healthy foot should be. Note how well formed the arch of the foot is. The dotted line indicates the condition of the foot of a person subject to fallen arches, also how the foot of a person looks who has flat feet. Note the bone construction of the foot in Fig. 2 and how Figs. 3, 4, and 6 show the ligaments and muscular construction of the foot. When these ligaments lose their muscular support they sag and allow the bones in the arch of the foot to drop. This condition causes innumerable physical and nervous ailments.

Fig. 7

The leg muscles need more muscular stimulation from exercise than the arms. Once the muscle tissues of the leg begin to break down they will build up as rapidly as any other muscle in the body. They become pliant, and powerful, and stored up in each separate muscle is a degree of untiring endurance hard to beat. But exercise alone will not provide endurance—there are other means I will discuss later. Sufficient is it that exercise provides the stuff endurance is made out of.

The nerves in your leg and its great arterial construction have a great deal to do with the quality of endurance in the legs. In the first place the muscles of the legs are the farthest removed from the heart, also they are the largest muscles in the body. Even though you may have a 16-inch pair of biceps and calves, you must not forget that in the arms the triceps supply one- fourth of the substance to provide a 16-inch biceps, but in the calf the circumference must come from the gastrocnemius alone. The thigh muscles easily outdo any of the body muscles in size.

The larger the muscles are the greater the supply of fuel they require, and this fuel is in the form of blood. The heart has to pump the supply to the muscles in large quantities, especially when under great physical strain. If the leg muscles are low in nerve vibration the arterial canals of the lower limbs will be sluggish and circulation impeded. The veins which carry away the impure blood will be choked with organic debris, all of which makes the refueling process very hard and strenuous upon the heart. Nature has conspired somewhat against us also in this case, inasmuch as in the legs, the blood flow rises contrary to gravity which requires more cardiac pumping than is necessary for the upper body muscles in order to give energetic function. Therefore, it can be readily understood that the arterial and vein canals must be stimulated and aided as much as possible without throwing any undue strain upon the heart. This done, greater nerve vibration follows, your muscles are made dynamic and blood replenishment flows evenly to all the muscles in the leg.

Another verv important organic condition takes place within the great bone of the lower leg which means considerable to your entire bodily health. Within the marrow of the shin bones are born the life blood corpuscles of the body. These corpuscles compose the nucleus of the blood stream. An abundance of red corpuscles in the body means a richer blood stream. They manifest that clean feeling of life within the veins with which those who are abundantly endowed with health are familiar. It is claimed at death these corpuscles are greatly diminished in the body. The marrow within the bones is starved so they cannot manufacture these life corpuscles in sufficient quantity. These life germs are thrown out through the porous sections of the bone into the blood stream and rely upon blood circulation to distribute them throughout the body to feed the muscles and organs. As you ponder over this the importance of leg development will be more impressed upon you—which is just what I wish to see.

I want you to remember that all muscles have direct nerve impulses and the best way to promote this is by a healthy, clean blood circulation gotten from common sense systematic progressive exercise. It is also well to remember that massage plays a very important part in muscular leg building. Not only will correct massage aid in breaking down the old tissue, but it will make the muscles more responsive, will help the nerve sources to reach out more vigorously, and will stimulate slow blood circulation into a thrilling, active life stream of superlative health.

The heel bone and the foot compose lever and fulcrum action and the shin bone by insertion into the ankle gives support. These three points are vital. Their qualities are manifested in balance in physical poise, and these can only be gotten from the sturdy well-balanced condition of your leg muscles.

Performing leg exercises while handling very heavy weight is suicidal. The depression on the upper body is far too much for the organs to stand. How can the heart pump fuel into the legs when the lungs are compressed and a congestion in the upper body blood channels is brought about from the strain? You know how hard it is to draw a pail of water up from a deep well that is almost dry. It is one long haul. Well, it would be much harder to accomplish it if at the same time you had a heavy burden loaded on your shoulders. This is a fitting example of the long haul the heart has in order to throw blood into the leg blood stream. It is made more difficult by the bodily resistance fighting the additional weight which many handle in exercise in order to get the required resistance from the leg muscles. The only way you can get satisfaction in leg development is to exclude exercises that cause muscular and organic strain on the upper body. The resistance must be centered and concentrated where it belongs and I will show you how that can be done safely.

There is an exercise greatly recommended among exponents of heavy exercise as good for the muscles on the back of the legs. Perhaps you are familiar with it. You lie flat on the back and balance a heavy weight on the soles of the feet and, by bending the knees, lower and push the weight up as the legs straighten on the knee. This exercise is very peculiar in its effect on the body. I used to practice it. First I started out with a light weight and noticed an unnatural change in the back. It started me thinking. I tried it several times and found my conclusions were right—then I quit. My conclusions were proved right later on by a young fellow who was a very promising featherweight strong man. He loved to practice this feat because he had very poor leg development—you'd know him if I mentioned his name. For some reason he began to get worse at lifting weights instead of better. He asked me the reason. I looked at his back and told him he would never be a successful lifter. I explained why, but he could hardly believe it until outraged nature proved it to him. He got so bad that he had to quit lifting and, finally forego the pleasure of exercising altogether. What happens is that the great depression caused by the weight forcing down compelled a bone change in the pelvis. The spine in the lower back region, instead of having the slight natural forward inclination, became straightened out so he could not bend his back in from the waist The back became straight all the way down from his shoulders. Now do not be confused by this statement and think it contrary to a natural straight back. The natural straight back is from the shoulder to the lumbar region, then, where the lumbar reeion meets the sacrospinalis, there is a slight tip forward so the hips set a little back to come squarely under the shoulders. This tip forward became thrown back so his hips were forward instead of a little back. In consequence he lost all control of equlibrium in lifting. Some who favor this exercise will try to prove their claim by saying the exercise is similar to the action of a "rizzly" performer—a man who lies on his back and juggles barrels on his feet and tosses them around. But this is not true. A "rizzly" performer when he lies on his back to perform does so on a specially made couch arrangement into which his hips fit so there can be no possible down pressure into the pelvis. You never see a "rizzly" performer handling a weight that forces his knees onto the sides of his body. He uses his leg muscles only. The objects he juggles are comparatively light for the leg strength he accumulates and his strength and leg development are gotten from continual practice and dexterity in handling the leg muscles only, in this performance. My life has been spent from an early age among athletes and performers and I have often practiced "rizzly" work and was quite expert in juggling a decent amount of weight on the feet in the position of the rizzly performer, so you see I speak from experience.

If you wish to practice this exercise, do so with a moderate weight. Better still, rig up a box with a hole in each side, into which tie a rope and have the box suspended from a rafter so that when the soles of the feet are fully supporting the box, the knees are at least a foot away from the floor when the knees are bent. See Fig. 8. You will then get the right leg muscle action for developing purposes and there will never be any danger of having the knees forced down on the body.

The object of the box is to provide you with more foot pushing space and give better balance

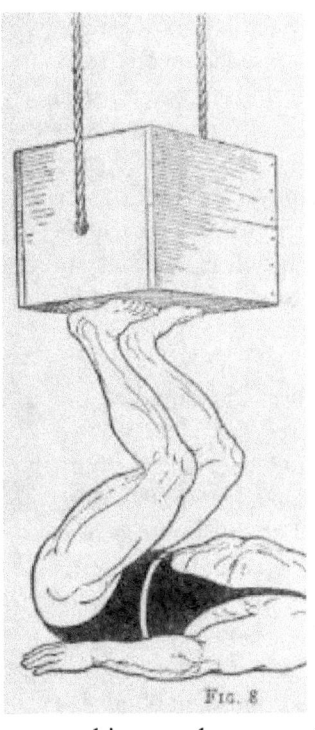
Fig. 8

and control. You can load the box with whatever amount of weight you wish to handle. It also removes the fear of the object rolling off the feet which often makes one nervous.

Men who have a pronounced inverted curvature from bending far back when pushing a weight overhead are never any good at handling objects in the "rizzly" position, neither is a man good at raising weight overhead in any position who consistently practices pushing up heavy weights on the feet without using the precautionary box method I have just mentioned.

In other words the leg press exercise, as they call it, is only good as I have explained. When practicing the leg press exercise place the palms of the hands flat on the floor, but under the side of each hip. You will be surprised how this will help you to better control the exercise and relieve the pelvis of even the slightest strain.

Good legs will always be the deciding factor of a man's physique and bodily power.

Equilibrium is controlled by the leg muscles and the gripping power of the toes adds greatly to it. This is proved by dancers, sprinters, jumpers, and men who are active on their feet. The slogan "Get on your toes" is no idle saying, but has originated from the fact that people, physically active and alert, are always up on their toes. You cannot spring from a flat-foot position. It is necessary to bound from the ball of the foot. Dempsey got all his tigerish attack from his ability to keep on his toes.

The foot and the leg form the tripod of life and as I explained before, from these two members are gotten fulcrum, lever and support. The leg arterial blood channels are the deep mainstays of your health. Let the flow become inactive and you begin to deteriorate. So let us exercise and get all the benefit we can out of these powerful members of our bodies.

And now let us see what manner of exercise we can devise that will make those stubborn leg muscles grow. The kind which you will enjoy and be able to practice without anv upper body strain. Also we want exercises that will give you plenty to work on and will give you satisfaction and a new zest for leg building.

EXERCISE ONE

CUP the hands on the hips standing perfectly erect. Space the feet apart just a few inches—enough to give you good balance. We will take the right leg first. The left leg must be kept locked at the knee throughout the entire movement. Raise the right leg directly forward pointing the foot like a dancer. (Position 1.) Without bending the right knee and postively without leaning back raise the right leg as high forward as you can. Remember the left leg must be straight all the time. When you feel you have raised the right leg as high as it will go, pause a moment and bend the foot on the ankle so it is at right angles to the leg. (Position 2.) As this foot movement takes place you will feel a strong pull on the muscles back of the thigh, particularly in the region behind the knee where the ligaments of the biceps insert. As you feel this pull, slowly bend the knee and point the toe to- war d s the floor, gradually bringing the knee up on the body. (Position 3.)

If you practice this exercise slowly and exactly as given here what will be felt will be a powerful extension and contraction of the thigh biceps muscles. As the thigh comes up on the body as much as possible—which will not be much—draw the heel up toward the buttocks. Keep the toes forcibly pointed down and you will call into play the gastrocnemius muscles. This movement completed, place the foot back on the floor and repeat the exercise as many times as you are comfortably able, then exercise the left leg in the same fashion.

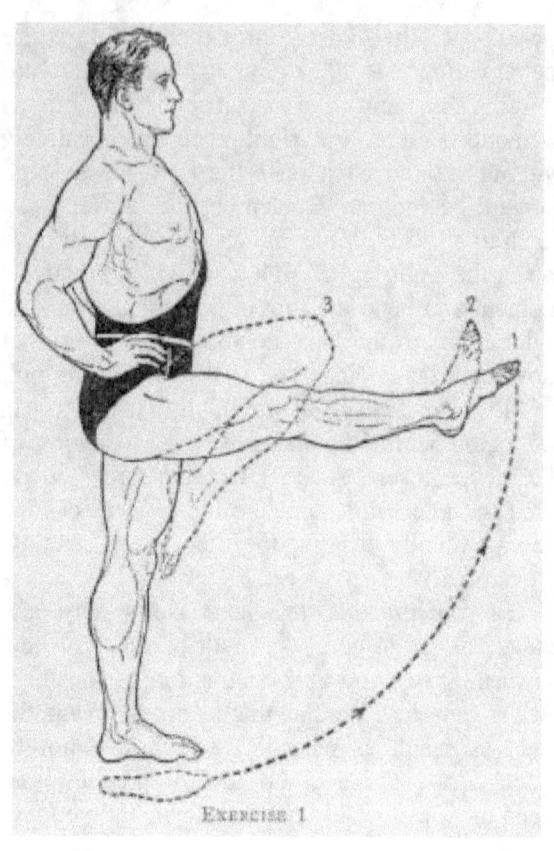

EXERCISE 1

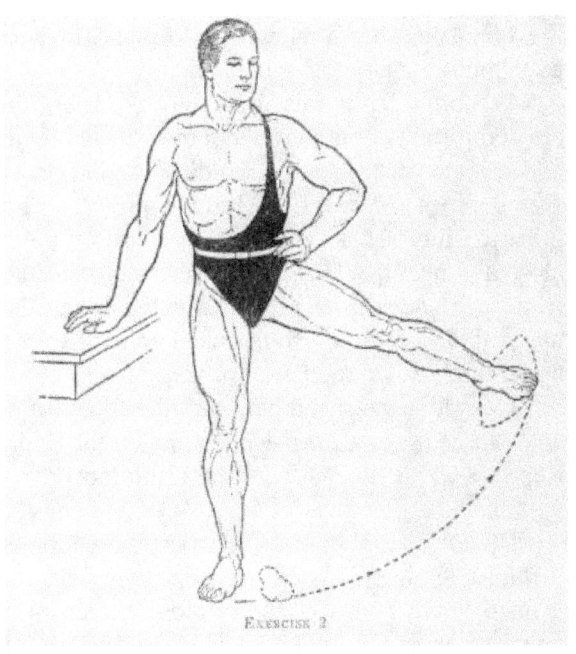

Exercise 2

EXERCISE TWO

This exercise is going to feel very awkward. You will find it difficult for a time to preserve your balance so to begin with I would advise you to stand near to the wall so you can help control your balance by placing your hand on the wall. Or you may place your hand on the table, bureau or on a chair back.

The object is to stand squarely upon one foot and raise the other leg out sideways as far as it will go without forcing you to lean too far over to the opposite side. You will be obliged to lean over slightly, but let it be only slightly.

When the leg is raised laterally as far as you are comfortably able, turn the foot on the ankle in and out all you can while holding the leg up to your limit in the lateral position. You will feel a great tension on the outside muscles of the thigh close to the hip. This is that muscle, separate from the quadriceps femorus, which fills out the upper thigh providing fulness and contour to the upper thigh called the tensor of fascia lata.

I would suggest that you turn the foot on the ankle three times, then place the foot on the floor. Repeat several times. Then repeat the movement with the other leg.

Do not worry about the number of repetitions for this exercise. You will not be able to perform it many times and it is one of those exercises in which it is not wise to let any set number of repetitions govern.

EXERCISE THREE

Very few ever get any results from practicing this exercise generally known as the "toe raise." If you compare Fig. 1 with Fig. 2 you will readily see the reason. The majority of exercisers just teeter up on to the toes, even when performing the exercise slowly. They will tell you they have to do so in order to preserve their balance. As an ordinary movement it is the natural thing to do; unfortunately, the ordinary predominates too much in our lives, and here, as elsewhere, the ordinary acts to our disadvantage.

In Fig. 1 the straight line drawn through the body shows quite well how far the body is carried forward from the line of centralization. If you will examine Fig. 2 you will see the body is so perpendicular the line passes perfectly through the central points producing perfect equilibrium. This poise carries the body weight back, away from the toes, making it impossible for a person to teeter on the toes—he compels the 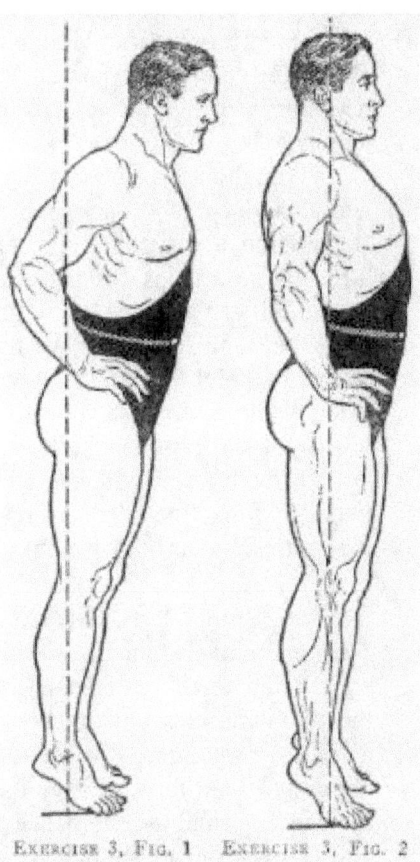 gastrocnemius muscles to lift the body weight. "This body lift" causes the lateral calf muscles to exert powerfully. The higher you are able to rise

EXERCISE 3, FIG. 1   EXERCISE 3, FIG. 2

on the toes, the more will you feel the lateral muscles tense in conjunction with the big twin calf muscles. You will feel the muscles that fit across the arch of the foot tighten. Sometimes this happens to such an extent, a cramp is felt in the arch of the foot. Do not let this worry you. It will do more good than harm. All you will find necessary to relieve it will be a little hand massage.

Throughout this performance keep the head and shoulders flung back, and the knees locked. If you find it difficult to preserve your balance allow the finger tips of one hand to rest lightly on a chair back. It will help you a great deal.

When you feel you have reached to the full extent of height upon the toes, lock the Imees forcibly and try to raise yourself some more.

If you do this exercise 12 to 18 times slowly, and correctly, you will be forever cured of the belief that the "toe raise" exercise is simple. The idea is to lift your body weight.

EXERCISE FOUR

This exercise is one that will be found very stimulating to the calf muscles and particularly the thigh muscles, but mostly the thigh biceps. That is, assuming you perform the exercise correctly. Bend forward from the waist and clasp the hands around the right knee. Lean forward all you can without losing balance and point the toe toward the floor. This done, begin to pull up with hands with all your power, at the same time resist the effort by exerting with the thigh muscles down. As you pull up with the hands, straighten the back to aid your arm power. Keep on pulling up until the thigh is forced upon the body as much as possible. But at no time allow the toe to deviate from the floor-pointing position. In fact accentuate this line of effort as the knee lift is in progress. Lift the heel toward the buttock. Get all the possible contraction into the exercise.

When you have finished this movement, relax. Unclasp the hands and place the foot on the floor, then repeat the exercise all over. When six repetitions have been done with the right leg then practice six times with the left leg, increasing the number of repetitions as you feel able.

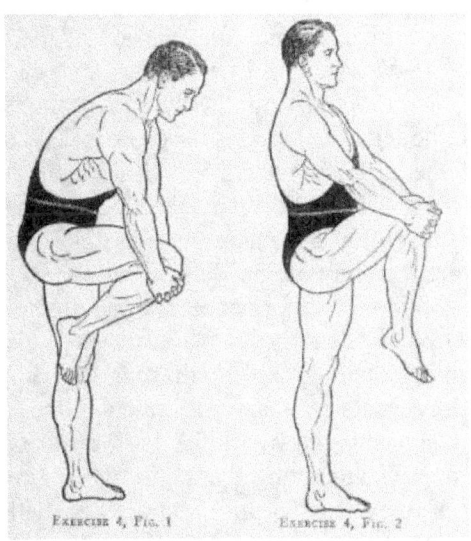

EXERCISE 4, FIG. 1   EXERCISE 4, FIG. 2

EXERCISE FIVE

Here is an exercise that you are going to find very awkward. When you have read the instruction you are going to figure it as being very simple but if you do find it simple you will have overlooked some very important points.

This exercise is particularly directed to the muscle that rises on the outside of the thigh above the vastus externus and to the sartorious and gracilis muscles.

The main object is to see that the movement is performed with the leg and not by the body. Cup the hands on the hips— not arms by sides. Raise the leg forward all you can without leaning back and without bending the supporting leg. When you feel the muscular tension of the thigh muscles you will have lifted the leg high enough. Now, without moving the body on the waist move the leg out sideways all you can; this done, move the leg back to the front position, but do not stop here; instead, move the leg across the supporting leg as much as possible without twisting the body on the waist. Keep the leg high throughout the performance and point the toes forward. In fact, the movement is similar to describing a half circle with the toes.

Only practice three movements one time, then change, giving the other leg exercise, then change back, directing the same total of repetitions in relay fashion until you are satisfied you have done enough.

EXERCISE SIX

This exercise calls into existence the force of opposites. It will tell you better than the most competent instructor that ever lived, how much you know about your leg muscles and their manner of functioning. Every single muscle from the hips down becomes employed. It is a somewhat difficult exercise, but one well worth mastering.

Stand erect with hands cupped on the hips, then step back with the right foot about a foot—although this distance is not definite. People with longer legs will be required to step back farther. A few practices will give you the right distance. Now strongly tense every muscle in the legs and begin to rise on the toes; as you do so, bend the knees, and force yourself forward in an endeavor to place both knees on the floor at the same time. Of course you will not be able to do so, nor does the exercise require that, but it does require that you must force yourself forward until the knees are about three or four inches off the floor. When this stage is gained, pause a moment and by exerting the muscles in the opposite direction come back to the erect position. Above all things, do not seesaw to and fro. It is a waste of time. Force yourself forward by strongly tensing the muscles and you will feel the splendid effects of this exercise all through the legs. Keep up on the toes. That part is very important. If you find it difficult to keep your balance with the hands cupped on the hips, use a chair in front of you.

Grip the chair back with one hand to maintain your balance.

After you have pressed forward with the left foot advanced, change. This time put the right foot forward, but remember, you must force yourself forward and down toward the floor.

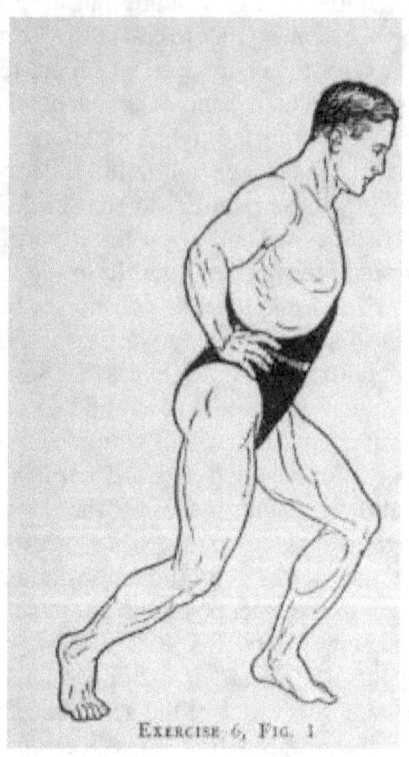

EXERCISE 6, FIG. 1

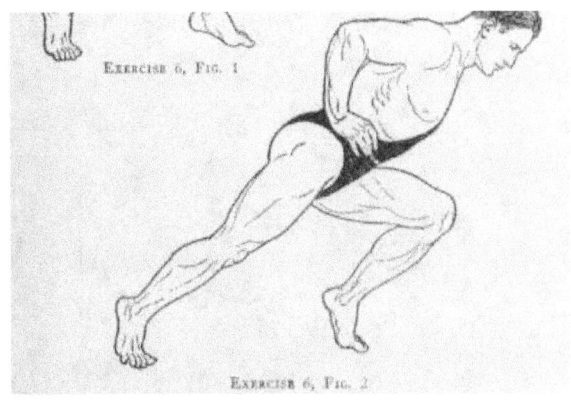

Exercise 6, Fig. 1

Exercise 6, Fig. 2

EXERCISE SEVEN

The reason why the ordinary "deep knee bend' exercise gives but little results is for much the same reason that the "toe raise" exercise fails—the average person is too familiar with performing the movement in the easiest way, and automatically they practice in that set groove. In this exercise I am changing the foot and knee positions in order to obtain different muscle volition. Not only will the varied character of this exercise keep your mind on it, but it will compel the sar- tonus and gracilius muscles to function strongly as well as the jemoralis and vastus externus muscles. The calf muscles and the ankles and knees come in for new action and it all helps.

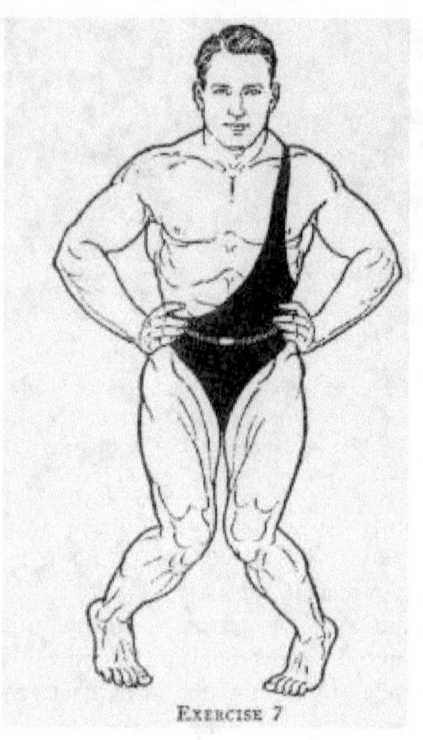

EXERCISE 7

Cup the hands on the hips, and stand with the feet ^ well apart and the toes turned in all you can. From this awkward position begin to bend at the knees and descend into a semi-sitting position. As you descend into the sitting position bring both knees forcibly together—not quickly, but slowly. In this position you will find it difficult to make the complete "squat," as we call sitting on the heels, but this is not necessary. If you practice this movement 18 times putting plenty of action into the knee-closing movement you will feel you have done enough. Still what I want to impress on you is action.

EXERCISE EIGHT

Assume the sitting position on the floor exactly as the figure in this exercise illustrates. Cross the arms placing the right hand against the inside of the left knee. Hold t\e knees fairly close together, and draw the heels up towards the seat. This done, get ready for the exercise.

With all your power push with each hand against the inside of the thigh and as you do so resist the pressure of the hands by squeezing in with the knees.

The object is to spread the knees apart all you can with your hands, resisting with your thigh force. When the knees have been spread apart all they will go, slip the hands across the knees so the fingers are pulling in on the knees. Forcibly try to pull the knees together with the hands and with the thigh resist the effort, but do not exert so much leg strength as to overpower the arm pull. Bring the knees together. This done repeat the first part of the exercise. In other words the first part of the exercise you push the knees apart and in the second stage you pull them together, but in each movement you resist with the legs.

This is a corking good exercise for the muscles along the inside and the outside of the thigh. It also helps materially in building up the shoulder and breast muscles.

51

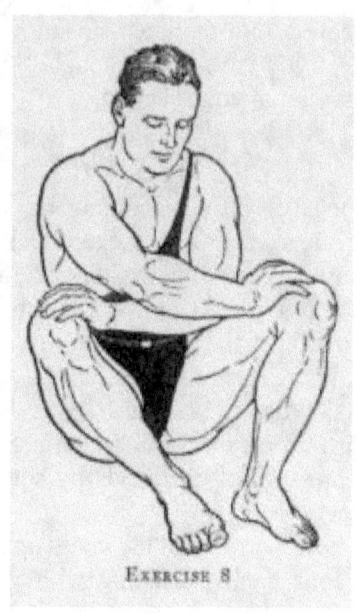

EXERCISE 8

EXERCISE NINE

Here is an exercise that will test how much lifting power your calf muscles have. If you notice carefully the position in the accompanying illustration you will see that this exercise is a combination of the toe raise and a lift. Actually it is not a lift. The apparent lifting position is purely a check to the power of the legs in raising up the body weight.

Stand close up to a very heavy bench or table. Place the hands under the edge in a lifting grip and bend the body slightly forward from the waist. Use just enough exertion to give you a strong up-pull on the table. This done, begin to raise yourself up on the toes slowly and forcibly. If the strength exerted in the toe-raise is sufficient to lift the body weight, and the weight of the table, all well and good, but you positively must not allow the strength of the body or the arm to help in the least the lifting up of the table. Maybe you will not be able to lift the table, but that does not matter, the effort supplied by the up-lift on the table will exert the calf muscles to an extraordinary degree. As you rise, do so squarely on the ball of the foot. Some people twist the foot so the pressure is borne mainly on the outside of the foot. This is entirely wrong, and minimizes the resistance of the calf muscles, particularly the

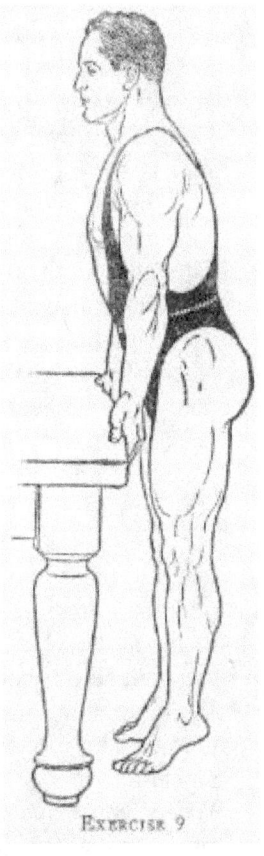

Exercise 9

gastrocnemius muscle. The greater part of the pressure should be borne on the inside of the foot by the great toe. Raise yourself as high on the toes as you can without bending the knees. You will find this exercise an interesting progression upon the ordinary toe-raise.

EXERCISE TEN

Take a towel or anything else similar that will answer the purpose, grasping an end in each hand. The towel will then form a loop. Place the foot in the loop, but see that only the ball of the foot rests in the loop. If you place the arch of the foot in it you might as well not do the exercise. The toes and the ball of the foot only must rest in the loop. Raise the knee high—higher than shown in the picture as that really depicts the halfway stage of the exercise. Point the toes all you can and carry the heel back towards the buttock. Not back all the way, just enough to give you strong gastrocnemius and thigh biceps tension and a good flexion of the knee. From this point begin the exercise. Keep the supporting leg stiff and begin to press down with the foot in the sling. As you press down resist the movement with the pull of the arms. That is, lift upon the foot. Keep the toe pointed all the time and force down until the leg is straight, and the muscles in the leg fully tensed. This done relax and draw the knee up repeating the forcing-down movement again. When you have performed with the one leg enough to suit yourself change over and give the other leg a workout. Do not be afraid to put plenty of pressure behind the foot movement or in the pull-up with the arms. That is where the value lies.

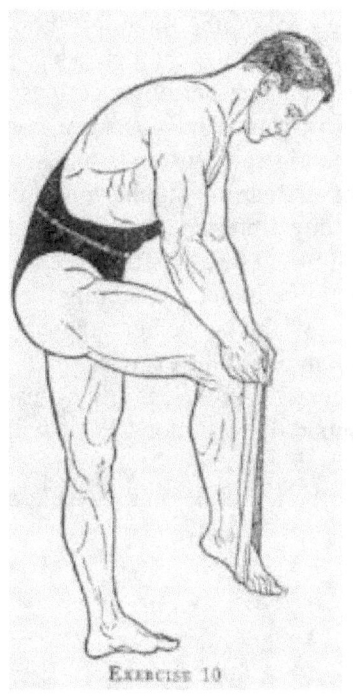

Exercise 10

EXERCISE ELEVEN

In this exercise you place the foot in the loop as
the illustration shows, with an end of the towel
held in each hand. The knee is carried somewhat
forward of the perpendicular line and the foot is
pulled up so that the distance between the heel
and the ankle is shortened. The object of the
exercise is not only to pull up on the towel and so
force the heel closer to the buttock, but, what is
more important, to pull the leg and the knee back

all it will go before the final operation of pulling the heel closer to the buttock takes place. The foot throughout the performance must be pulled up all it will stand and you must contract very strongly the big calf muscle, also resisting all the up-pull of the arms pulling on the loop, by exerting a down pressure with the thigh muscles. The farther back you allow the knee to travel, and the closer to the buttock you bring the heel at the conclusion of the movement the greater value will be gotten out of the exercise.

Practice with both legs giving each leg the same number of repetitions. You will find it a corking good exercise for the ankle and calf, knee, back thigh muscles and the buttock.

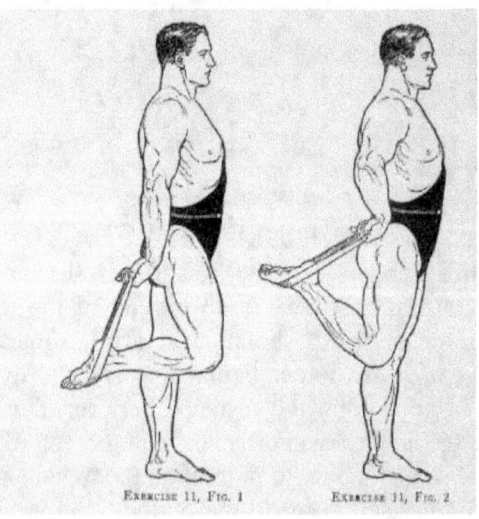

EXERCISE 11, FIG. 1   EXERCISE 11, FIG. 2

JOWETT INSTITUTE OF PHYSICAL CULTURE,
SCRANTON, PA.

Dear Mr. Jowett:

I am deeply interested in getting a body like yours. I want health, strength, endurance, nerve energy and vital life and would appreciate your sending me free of any obligation on my part your big illustrated book, "The Thrill of Being Strong," which will explain how I can get all these physical treasures.

Name _____ Age _____

Address _____

_____

216

JOWETT INSTITUTE OF PHYSICAL CULTURE,
SCRANTON, PA.

Dear Mr. Jowett:

I am deeply interested in getting a body like yours. I want health, strength, endurance, nerve energy and vital life and would appreciate your sending me free of any obligation on my part your big illustrated book, "The Thrill of Being Strong," which will explain how I can get all these physical treasures.

Name _____ Age _____

Address _____

_____

58